The Magic of Bananas

For Cooking and Healing

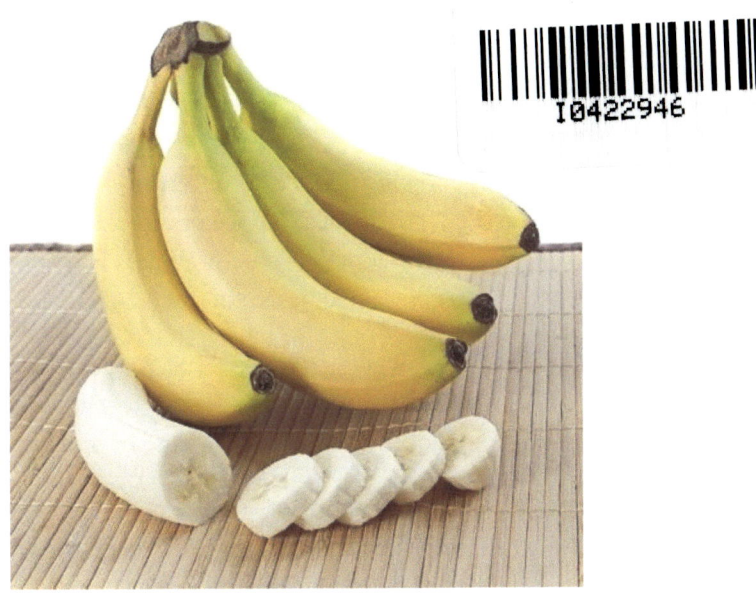

By Dueep Jyot Singh

Natural Remedy Series

Mendon Cottage Books

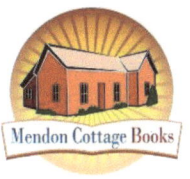

JD-Biz Publishing

Disclaimer

The information is this book is provided for informational purposes only. It is not intended to be used and medical advice or a substitute for proper medical treatment by a qualified health care provider. The information is believed to be accurate as presented based on research by the author.

The contents have not been evaluated by the U.S. Food and Drug Administration or any other Government or Health Organization and the contents in this book are not to be used to treat cure or prevent disease.

The author or publisher is not responsible for the use or safety of any diet, procedure or treatment mentioned in this book. The author or publisher is not responsible for errors or omissions that may exist.

Warning

The Book is for informational purposes only and before taking on any diet, treatment or medical procedure, it is recommended to consult with your primary health care provider.

Our books are available at

1. Amazon.com
2. Barnes and Noble
3. Itunes
4. Kobo
5. Smashwords
6. Google Play Books

Download Free Books!

http://MendonCottageBooks.com

Table of Contents

Introduction

If you were a part of the flapper scene in the roaring 20s and 30s you would be Charleston-ing to "Yes, yes, we have no bananas." "Going bananas" was popular slang for someone who thought he or she was losing his marbles over someone or something. A Bright Young Thing of that Era would tell her "Sheik" that she considered him to be the bee's knees , and the cat's pajamas and she was going bananas over him, but … if he was found escorting any other "Sheba" around to trip the light fantastic, she would have his blood for breakfast.

So what is there in this not so humble plant, which makes it such an integral part of popular culture, as well as slang? Well, firstly, bananas are delicious treats to have throughout the day. Also, they are rich in potassium and other minerals, which keep you fit and fine and glowing and chirpy. Also, the name is rather amusing, so no wonder the whole world has gone bananas over bananas. Since millenniums, the economies of countries have depended upon this delicious fruit.

You can eat these bananas and raw or you can need them ripe. You can roast them, fry them, boil them, mash them, and then your imagination is the limit to which particular use, you want to put these bananas.

Bananas are normally eaten raw, but when you decide to cook them, you are going to choose bananas called plantains with more starch content. They may be raw bananas.

The color of our banana ranges from green to yellow. You may also have brown, red, and purple bananas depending on the species and the state of ripeness.

The bananas were called Musa sapientum by scientists before, but that name has now gone out of use. The banana species which we eat now belong to Musa balbisiana and Musa acuminata. Hybrids are also very popular, especially when Musa balbisiana is crossed with M.acuminata.

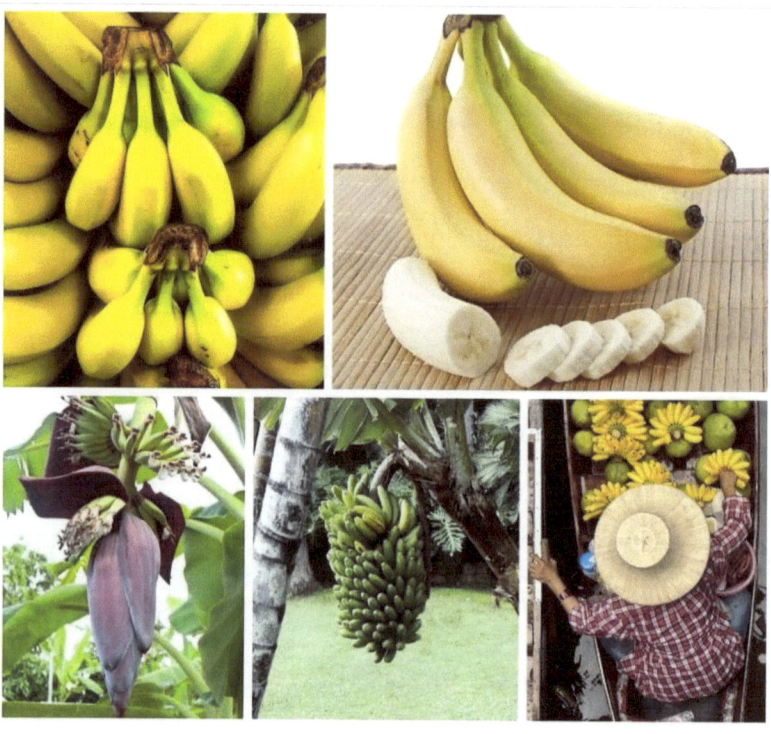

Most of the banana plants, which you find now are completely seedless. That is why if you are looking for seeds, to grow your bananas in your garden, sorry, you will need to plant a banana seedling, propagated by horticulturalist and gardeners.

Bananas are native to tropical Southeast Asia, the Indian subcontinent, Malaya and other tropical regions, as well as Australia. They grew wild in the tropical forests here until people started growing them in New Guinea anywhere between 5000 to 8000 years ago. From there, they spread all over the world.

Knowing More about the Banana

Egyptian papyri , going back more than 1200 years ago describe the glory of the banana. So that means it was cultivated extensively, there along with other regions of North Africa and the Middle East, in areas where there was plenty of water and sun around.

In fact this banana is such a precious fruit in the Oriental region of Asia, that I am reminded of an old ancient traditional folk story. This story is from Thailand.

Once upon a time, there was a man, who was considered to be the laziest mutt in the village. He kept on dreaming that he would be a multimillionaire, one day. But he made absolutely no effort to do something towards it. His wife sweated the whole day long so that her family could survive while her husband lay under a banana tree and dreamed of the glorious things he would do tomorrow.

One day, the wife's uncle came to their village to celebrate with his family on some festive occasion. He soon found out that the man was lazy to the bone, and a slacker. But as he happened to be very prosperous, the man stuck to him closer than glue.

"Oh, uncle, do tell me, what made you so rich? Do you have some magical formula which made all this come to pass? Something which does not need hard work?" Said the slacker in admiring tones.

"Well, this is a secret, but as you are my niece's husband, I am going to give you this secret. But for that, you would need some very special magic. And that magic can only be obtained when you get me 5 kg of the white powder that you collect from the under portion of the banana leaves grown in your garden. Take care of all those banana plants, after you have planted them in your own garden by your own hands. And do not tell anyone this secret ever. "

This was magic! Naturally, the man immediately requested his neighbors to give him as many plants as they could spare. He needed just banana plants.

The very next morning found him planting his garden with magic banana plants. He tended them like he would tend treasures, because after all these plants were going to make him very, very rich. All the magic was under the leaves of the bananas, and he was very happy to see them grow and flourish.

The only problem was that the powder under the leaves was so small in quantity, but he persevered. It would take him years and years to complete uncle's order of the magic powder, but he intended doing just that.

The bananas grew, and they began to fruit. The wife collected the fruit, and began to sell it in the market. But her husband was interested in just the powder under the leaves. Within a couple of years, the wife who was a good businesswoman made quite a good living, thanks to the banana crop. Besides, her husband kept on replenishing the bananas which had died or grown old, with new bananas planted by his own hands and fed and watered.

40 years later, the man managed to collect 5 kg of magic banana powder and took it to the wise old uncle, who was still alive.

"Well, my son, thank you for the powder." Said the uncle and threw it all in the river!

The horrified man shrieked with astonishment and horror. He had spent 40 years of his life collecting that precious powder and the uncle had thrown it in the river?

"Well, that was my magic, my son. It was this river, which was loaded with the bananas from your garden, and which took those boats to cities far away from here. And the river brought back the profits made from those sales. So do not you see how the magic worked, with the powder off the backs of these banana leaves?"

The moment I finished reading this story, I went right to my garden, and inspected the banana leaves to see the white powder. I was all of eight years old at that time. I wiped a curious finger under the leaf. The powder barely covered my finger.

40 years, collecting that white powder patiently, year after year!

My immediate thought was oh, boy, these adults are crazy! What would they not do for money?

But then, this is an ancient story and practical children are not known for their patience.

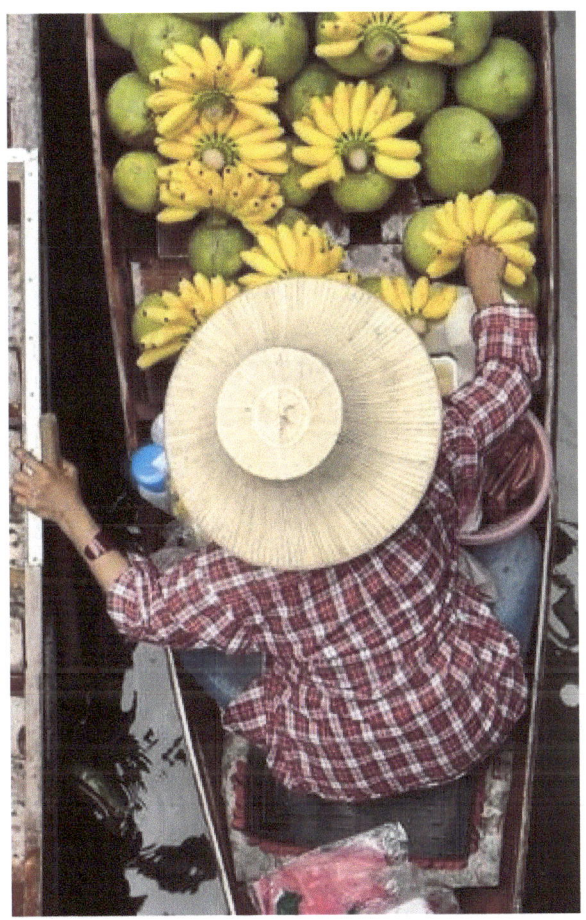

21st century Floating market in Thailand, on the water, and with bananas being very much a part of it!

Bananas, believe it or not, are the fourth most important food crop of the world. In fact, bananas are considered to be a complete food. So anyway, you do not see wheat, rice, or corn growing, the important cash crop to feed the multitudes will be bananas.

Portuguese traders were instrumental in taking the bananas to the Americas, in the 15th and 16th centuries, where they flourished. Plantations of Barbados and Jamaica prospered on sugarcane and bananas. In fact, anybody who remembers that Calypso song " Day-O" is going to remember those words,

Come, Mister Tally Man, tally me banana
(Daylight come and me wan' go home)
Come, Mister Tally Man, tally me banana
(Daylight come and me wan' go home)

Lift six foot, seven foot, eight foot bunch
(Daylight come and me wan' go home)
Six foot, seven foot, eight foot bunch
(Daylight come and me wan' go home)

These bananas collected from these plantations would then be shipped all over the world.

Growing Bananas

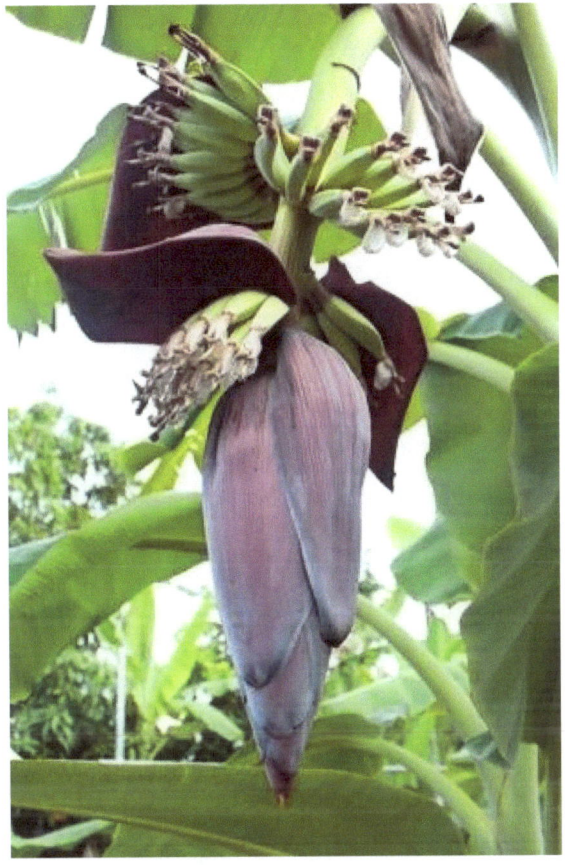

Banana tree with purple flower and green fruit. Remove the purple portion, after the fruit has begun to make an appearance.

Bananas can be grown very easily in well-drained soil. Make sure that there is no stagnation, water collected around the roots are going to cause root rot. Too much water only broadens the leaves, and grows more tubers.

The banana tree is perennial, so once you have planted the rhizome or the bulb, you just need to take care of it, so that it can grow well.

Once the fruit starts growing on the stem, which is going to be within a year of planting, with the flower appearing within six months, they are ready to harvest.

Best Temperature for Bananas

Bananas flourish in areas where the average temperature is 27°C and the rainfall is up to 80 – 98 inches. That is why they are grown extensively in tropical climates, where there is plenty of sun, the winters are not harsh, and the rain is also plentiful. So if you are around the equator, you are going to see plenty of bananas growing there.

Preparing the Ground for Bananas

Bananas have been known to grow up to 25 feet! So you have to make sure that the areas in which you plant them, give them plenty of elbow space to grow, both sideways and upwards. That is because the leaves are going to take up plenty of space when mature.

Many times people looking at bananas for the first time, thinking that they are trees, even though the stems are not woody. The stems are called pseudostems and are green in color.

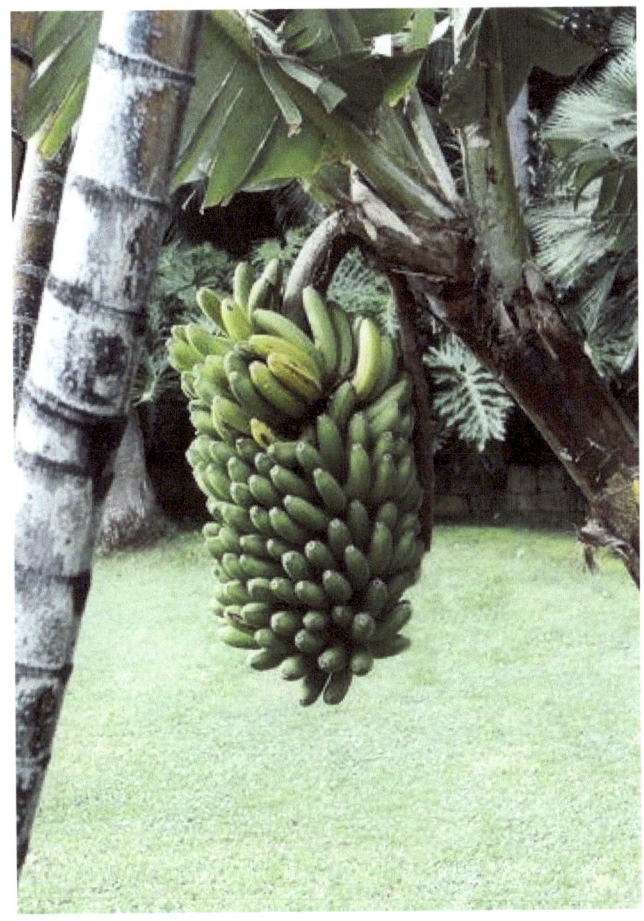

Bananas are best grown in the sun so that the leaves can gain benefit from the direct sunlight. Also, the soil needs to be warm, and that is why bananas do not flourish in lands, where the winters are harsh and frosty. If the soil temperature is around 20°C throughout the year, you are going to have healthy and happy bananas.

So while picking the best site, look for the place where you get the most sun. You can also grow them in pots and in greenhouses, as long as you have plenty of space for future banana growth.

Banana Growing Tips

It is much more sensible not to crowd banana plants together. If you do so, you are going to have a competition about which plants can manage to garner more nutrients from the soil, thus stunting the growth of other plants. So if you really want to grow lots of banana plants, make sure that the distance between them is between 7 to 8 feet.

Strapped for space? Try the dwarf varieties of which Cavendish is very popular. You can grow Cavendish in pots with a depth of 26 to 32 inches.

Planting Bananas

The well moisturized and well fertilized bed should be dug up properly, and the depth of the hole should be 30 cm. The diameter should be around 50 cm to fit the banana plant. Add organic fertilizer, to the soil, if you want.

Best is, of course, organic fertilizer, but chemical fertilizers are also much used, because farmers do not want to go through the trouble to find places where they can get pure organic fertilizer like leaf and bark compost, farmyard manure and other natural nutrients for healthy and natural plant growth.

Make sure that the organic fertilizer or the chemical fertilizer is not too much in quantity, because the roots of the banana are very delicate and can get burned.

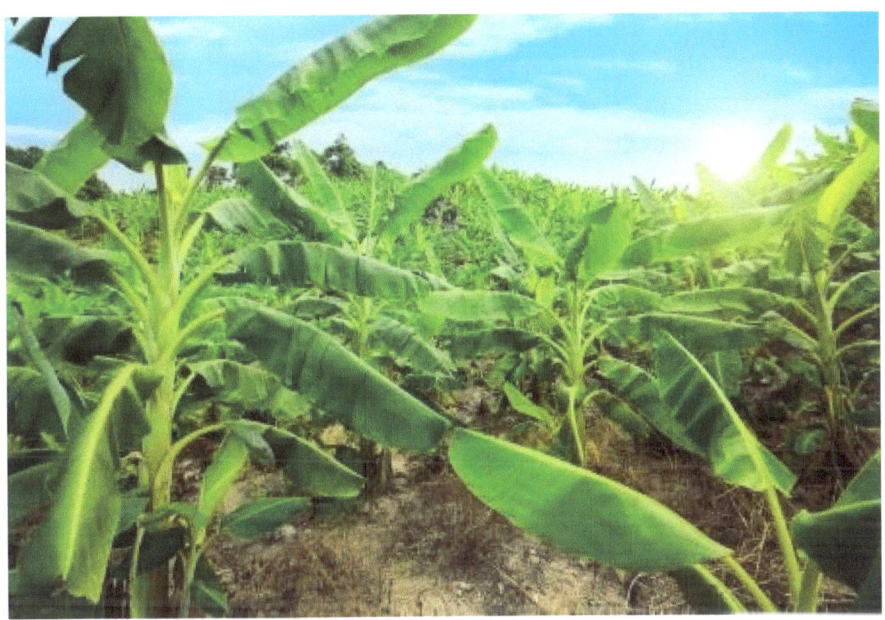

The small healthy shoot/sucker from the mother plant is going to be collected and planted elsewhere.

Why Not Seeds?

Sadly, banana fruit with seeds have grown extinct, down the ages and that is why you are either going to get a banana sucker from a nursery, or from your friends. The sucker should be between 1 feet to 4 feet high, with leaves already growing.

Use a sharp implement to separate this sucker from its mother banana plant. Do this very carefully. After that, you need to water and fertilize the mother plant, and refill the hole so that the mother plant does not start to lean because it has lost the support of the sucker.

Nowadays, you can get tissue cultured plants, which yield higher bunches of bananas. They can be obtained on the Internet.

The roots of the sucker need to be trimmed until there are only about a couple of inches of roots. These routes are going to grow as soon as you plant them. Also remove any dried leaves or cut leaves. Your tree sucker should have 4 to 6 good and healthy leaves. That means all of the leaves are going to get plenty of sun, which also allows for the soil to dry up. Too many leaves means no sunlight passing through, and soil remaining moist for a longer period of time.

Place your banana plant in your already prepared and fertilized hole and make sure that it is standing upright as you fill in the hole. Tamp the soil down firmly, and then water it.

Remember not to water the plant daily if there is some water standing. Let the soil absorb the moisture, and as soon as it is dry, add some more water.

Fertilizer

Compost Is Definitely the Best Organic Fertilizer

Bananas need to be fed organic fertilizers once a month. Bananas are rich in potassium as well as in vitamins and that is why they need plenty of nutrients, which they are going to get from the organic soil.

If the temperature is not around 20°C for at least three fourth of the year, you need to compromise with feeding your plants with organic fertilizer so that they can grow well and get bananas ready for harvest in time.

You may also use old banana plants, which have been removed from your garden as chopped up Mulch. This is extremely good fertilizer, which is going to return a large quantity of potassium back to the soil. This green mulch can also be mixed up with other organic compost and mulch like Bracken, seaweed, and leaves. Adding too much fertilizer is definitely not recommended. Like I said before, that is going to burn the roots.

Banana Diseases

Bananas like other plants are also subject to a large number of diseases, which include root rot and bunchy top. Bananas in the Panama area suffer from Panama disease.

You can prevent this infection from spreading by removing all the infected leaves, and uprooting the infected plants. You will have to destroy them, so that the infection does not spread to the rest of the plants.

The moment your bananas begin sprouting, cut off the flower, so that they are allowed to grow unhindered.

The banana flowers of many South Asian varieties are edible, but others are totally inedible. So if you want to experiment with the banana flowers in your cuisine, checkup whether you can eat the flowers!

Ripening on the Tree

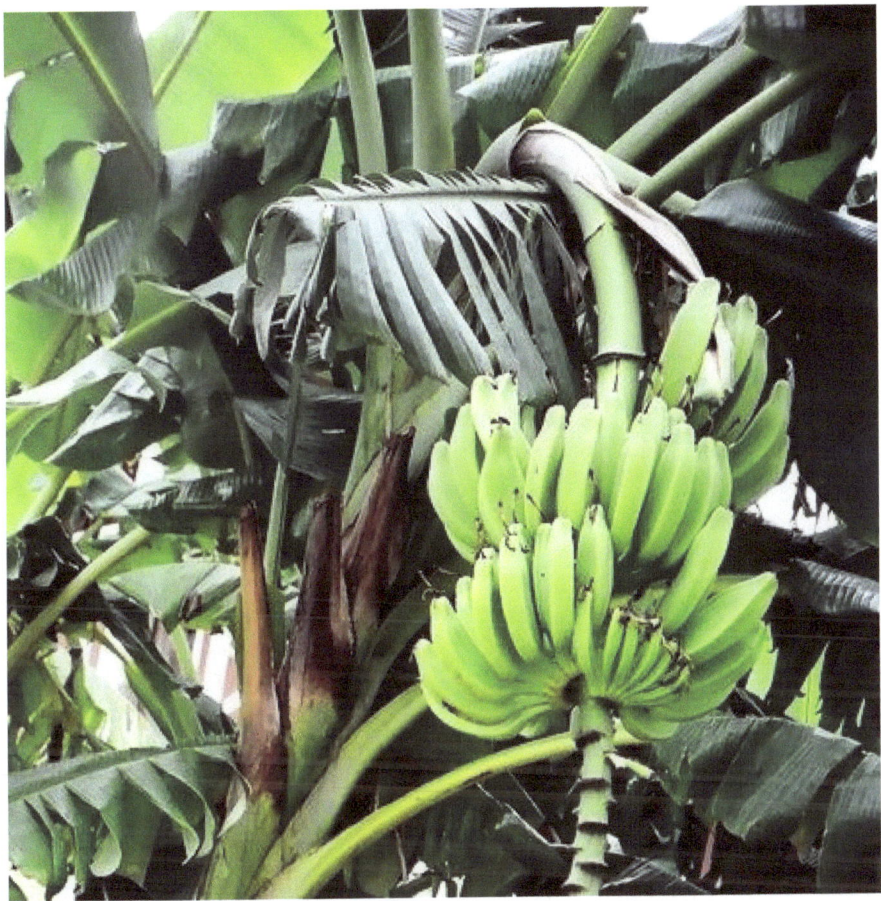

For best results, you need to make sure that the fruit ripens on the plant itself. The bunch should be harvested only when the skin turns a light orange in color. With time, and still on the stalk, this color is going to write on, the skin is going to get in there, and the inside of the banana berry is going to get pulpy.

Bananas ripened on the trees have a very limited shelf life. That is why many banana growers have the tendency to pluck the bunch of raw bananas, because after all, they are exporting them, and the time taken before the bananas reach their final destination is going to be enough, for the bananas to ripen. Artificial ripening processes include the use of chemicals, like carbide and other chemicals like ethylene oxide in airtight rooms.

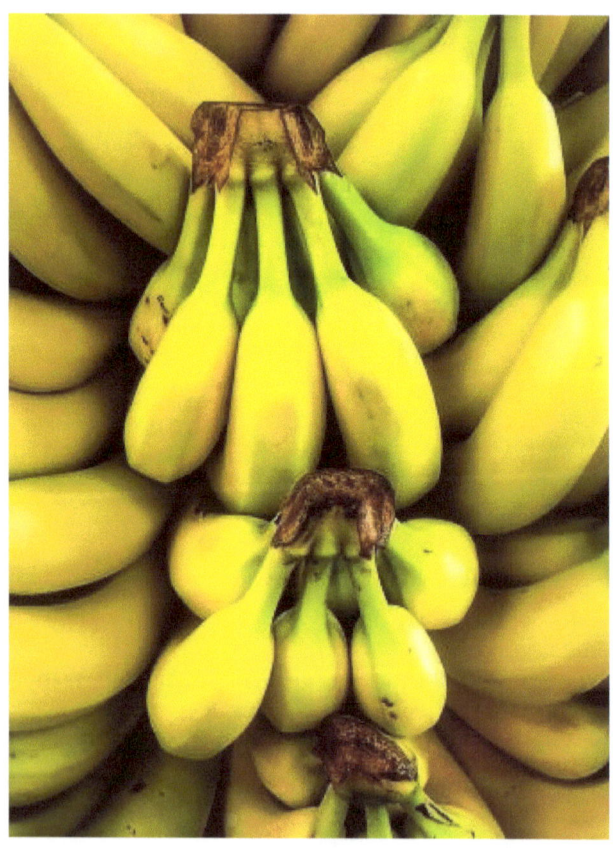

These bananas have been ripened artificially. See the green?

So how do you recognize that your banana has been artificially ripened? If the banana is green at its ends, but yellow in the middle, it was gathered from the tree, long before its time.

Instead, look for bananas, which are yellow, with small black patches. Press the fruit gently. They must give way. On the other hand, they should not have an overripe odor. That means they have passed their ripening time and are going to cause you problems in your tummy.

In fact, there is a Chinese variety, Go Sang Heong which can be literally translated into "the fruit that you can smell over the mountain!" It is sweet, delicious, and has a very fragrant aroma. Ripe bananas also have a mild aroma and overripe ones frankly smell!

The moment bananas begin to grow on your tree, you are going to be in competition with birds, squirrels, and even bats for first attack on these delicious fruit. So you can use the old ancient practice of covering the bunch with rice sacks. In the East, jute rice sacks are commonly used, but you can also use plastic sacks.

Cover this bunch, when it has aged for about two months. Make a hole in the bottom, so that the sack, which is acting like your greenhouse is well aerated, drained and kept warm. Also, the ripening fruit are going to produce ethylene oxide, which held in the ripening process. These fruit ripened naturally are the best bananas, you can gift to you and your family.

Harvesting Bananas

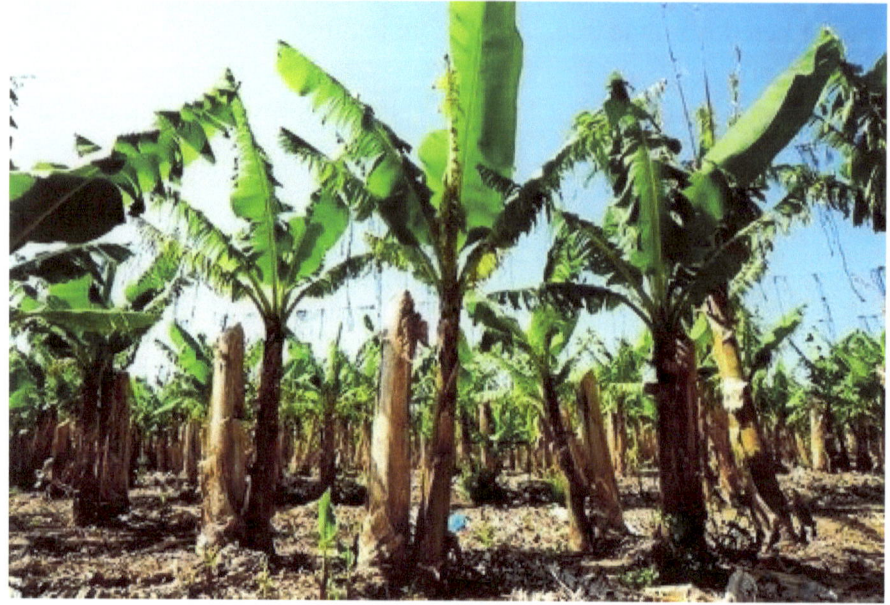

This is what your plantation is going to look like, after the fruit have been gathered. The plants are going to grow again from the mother stem.

The bananas are ready for harvesting about 2 ½ months, after you have covered them. One is going to know that because the leaves are going to die off. When there are about five still alive leaves on the plant, get ready to harvest.

Put on your well stained gardening sweatshirt, because a little bit of banana sap here and there, is not going to matter any. The sap of the banana, is definitely very difficult to remove, even with continuous washing.

Traditional harvesting is done by cutting a notch into the tree, on the opposite side of the fruit bunch. The stem is going to bend and you can thus gain easy access to the fruit. Cut the bunch off.

Do not worry about the cut portion. The tree is going to heal itself.

Remember that the shelf life of these bananas is rather less that is why you need to harvest them, only when you are ready to either ship them, transport them or eat them.

Bananas grown in pots are extremely attractive additions into your rooms, which provide a very good alternative to other foliage plants like Canna.

Storing of Bananas

The skins of Bananas stored in your refrigerator are going to turn into a black mass, due to the moisture. But I have not seen that having any effect on the fruit inside. Nevertheless, you should store bananas outside, in the fresh air, wrapped up in pieces of paper, so that they do not begin to over ripen.

I normally place them on top of the fridge so that I can get easy access to them whenever I am feeling hungry, and also to remind me to finish them before they turn overripe and fruit flies come visiting.

One Banana or Two?

Now let me tell you something interesting about bananas. Eat just one banana, and you may suffer from constipation. On the other hand, two bananas are considered to be the best way in which you can stay healthy, and also heal tummy problems.

I know about a family friend, who suffered terribly from ulcers. My father took him to lunch one day, and was surprised to see him stoking on bananas and nothing else. That was his lunch. He also said that this kept his stomach problem within controllable limits. Father saw him eating six – eight ripe bananas and following it up with water.

This problem cured itself within six months, thanks to the banana for lunch diet.

So here are some traditional medicines, which I am going to tell you in which you are going to eat two bananas.

Yogurt and Bananas

This is an extremely healthy combination. You can enjoy just as it is, or if you want to get a natural healer.

To heal any infections in your stomach – try two bananas, mashed up in a bowl full of fresh organic yogurt. Have this for lunch. Not only is it going to cure any infection, but it is an excellent way in which you can cure cramps in your tummy, as well as diarrhea.

Dry Cough

Take a banana skin, and cut it into small pieces. Dry it in the shade. You can also get powdered banana skin from beauty shops. Now roast this on the griddle, and then grind it, finely. Take one teaspoonful of this powder with 1 teaspoon of honey, twice a day. Believe it or not, this is a time tested ancient remedy to get rid of chronic cough. The banana skin heals the chest infection and the honey moisturizes your throat and prevents irritation.

Want to Gain Weight?

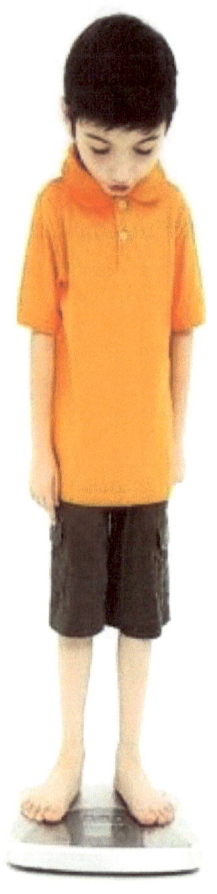

Too skinny and possibly suffering from bad eating habits.

Definitely not healthy.

In this world when everybody wants to be pencil thin and size 0, it is definitely not fashionable to have this bit of extra weight. Says who?

Spend a miserable youth and adulthood like mine with a terribly thin and lanky awkward totally flat and unshapely frame, where one couldn't gain weight, however much one ate. Good athletic muscle tone helps some, but it does not make you gain weight.

I spent my school and university years being called " Hey, Skeleton" or "Listen, Single Backbone". This androgynous Twiggy look is considered extremely attractive and desirable in the West and is the one to which a large number of teenagers aspire, but it is definitely looked askance in the East, where the feminine idea of beauty is 44 – 36 – 44. Besides, starving yourself to get that sort of shape like Victoria Beckham is definitely not a healthy state of mind or of body.

22 – 24 – 22 definitely did not come in that range! Of course, I had the frame for which models would happily murder me, without even bothering to diet or cutting down on butter, cream, and other delicious things which make life so worth living, including rich calorie and cholesterol laden food.

But from a normal red-blooded teenager and adult's perspective, this idea of staying a skeleton was terribly unappealing.

Until I was given some advice by the white witch of the town, the old herbal woman, who is the source of many of my herbal traditional and ancient remedies.

"Take two ripe bananas and then drink a glass of warm milk, for breakfast every day. Do this for two months. You will soon begin to gain weight."

I followed this, and began to look marginally human with a little bit of healthy weight in about 1 ½ months.

So if you want to put on some weight – whether you are male or female – try this. Guaranteed effective and guaranteed to work, unless of course, you suffer from inherited no weight genes- like I did – or any inherited chronic problem, which prevents you from gaining weight.

Ulcers in your mouth?

This normally happens when you suffer from constipation or when you have some other digestive problems. Just take yogurt with a teaspoonful of honey and two bananas, to cure your ulcers and your tummy problems.

Nosebleed

Nosebleed is not a common occurrence in places, where you are not subjected to sunshine in the high 35s during summer. Nevertheless, if you suffer from nosebleeds often, and you do not know how to get rid of them, take one ripe banana, and add some jaggery or molasses to it. Mash and drink with one glass of milk for a week. You are going to find you healed of any tendency to nosebleed unless someone punches you accidentally on the nose.

The Difference between Bananas and Plantains

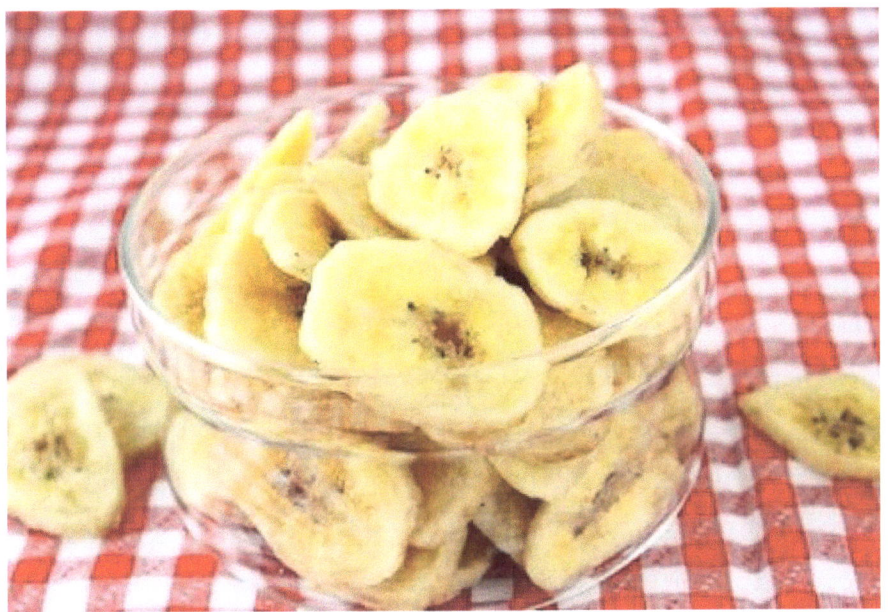

Plantains are starchy bananas, which can be used just like potatoes, especially in making banana chips.

I remember as a child getting into an argument with a friend, over the fruit that we were eating for lunch. I called them bananas and she called them plantains. Both of us persisted that the names taught to us by our parents was the right term. It was only more than three decades down the line, that I found out that plantains and bananas were synonymous.

It only depended on where you were in the corner of the globe. In the east, if you find a green starchy banana, which is normally used for cooking, you will call them plantains. In Europe, as well as in the Americas, bananas are used to describe the yellow pulpy sweet fruit, which you love eating raw, or in salads and in desserts in banana cookies, banana cakes, and other banana-based delicacies.

This distinction is only in English; the local vernacular term for bananas is going to be the word which has been used traditionally through generations.

It is surprising to know that bananas were not very well known in Europe, even up to Victorian times, with this much improved methods of locomotion, and it was Jules Verne , who described this fruit in his book around the world in 80 days, where he talked about Mr. Fogg encountering this fruit, during his travels in Asia.

However, thanks to modern transportation methods like steamships and rails, bananas from Caribbean countries began being exported to Europe.

Talking about Banana Republics

Heard the term banana republic? This is the 20th century term used to describe countries like the Honduras, of which the economic was completely relying on bananas. This economy was export-oriented. It did not contribute anything to the internal economic state or condition of the country. Many South and Central American countries began to be called banana republics, when Western companies importing bananas from them began to manipulate political factions, which would mean added profits to them.

The UK- exporting bananas from their Caribbean colonies – and the US – especially the United fruit Company, which is now well known globally as Chiquita- were main players in the setting up of these banana republics, with the political puppets of that country dancing to their piping.

This is because they knew, even in the late 19th and 20th century, that bananas were a major factor in world economic and trade, and those who had access to bananas, would be able to dictate political terms in places where these plants were both a part of economy, and also a part of survival.

Well, this manipulation is definitely a modern twist to the wars fought between European countries to gain access to and monopoly over the spice routes to Asia.

It is only in the Caribbean countries of which Dominica and Jamaica stand foremost – where they are producing enough of bananas for foreign export to North America and to Europe. In countries like India, as well as some other countries in Asia, and also some countries in Africa, the bananas are consumed within the local markets, grown and consumed locally.

That is because extensive banana cultivation and farming is not possible in places where the land is subjected to periodic typhoons and hurricanes. One teeny-weeny hurricane is going to reduce the whole year's banana crop to future mulch.

The most popular export bananas is the dwarf Cavendish because they are easy to transport, and their shelf life is longer.

Bananas as a Healthy Complete Food

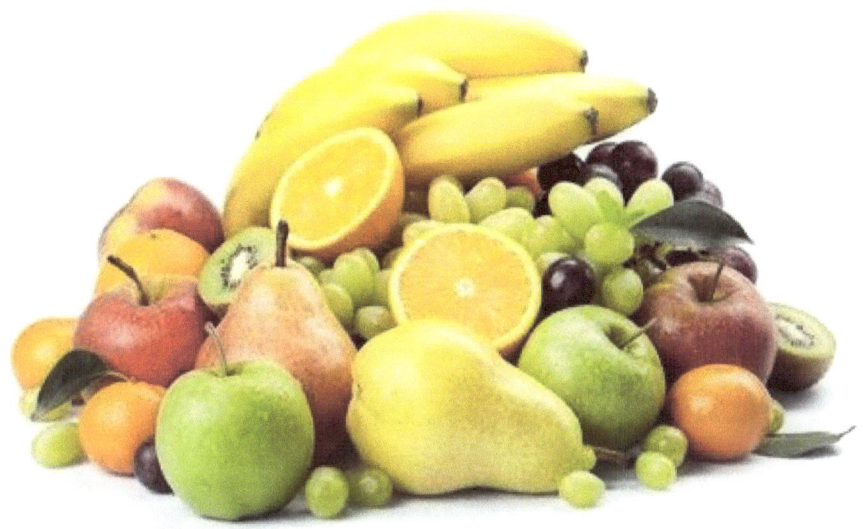

Bananas are top of the heap, to keep you healthy.

Some years ago, news channels were very excited about the discovery of an old Japanese soldier, who took to the forests after The Second World War because he was ashamed of the condition to which his proud country was reduced. This man survived for 40 years, on bananas and forests produce.

Well, he just proving the adage is that a banana is a major food and staple crop, which can be eaten cooked or ripe. Millions would agree with him, because they are surviving on bananas. They can grind these dried bananas and make them into a baking flour.

These bananas are starchy, and they can be boiled, fried, chipped, and baked just like potatoes and are almost as delicious. One banana is going to have about the same amount of calories which you are going to abstain from eating one potato.

It is said during the Second World War, that those prisoners who stayed in concentration camps where they got better access to bananas, were comparatively healthier, than those rescued from concentration camps where the fruit and vegetable content was minimal.

This is because these bananas are a really good source of potassium, manganese, vitamins B6 and also vitamin C.

There is only one thing you cannot get from bananas. That is banana juice! The moment you put it into your blender, you are going to get a pulp. So the best thing is, mix it in yogurt and drink it as a milkshake!

Banana Leaves

Traditionally, banana leaves have been used as a waterproof medium when still green. I remember sheltering under a wide banana leaf, when I was a kid, and as usual, got caught in a downpour. That is why these banana leaves are extremely popular, as eco-friendly and waterproof plates on which foods are served in many parts of Asia. In fact, the large leaves are used as umbrellas in many southeastern countries, even today.

Now serving food on banana leaves is also an interesting ancient tradition. You wash your hands and feet, and if you are eating your meal traditionally, you are going to sit cross legged on the ground.

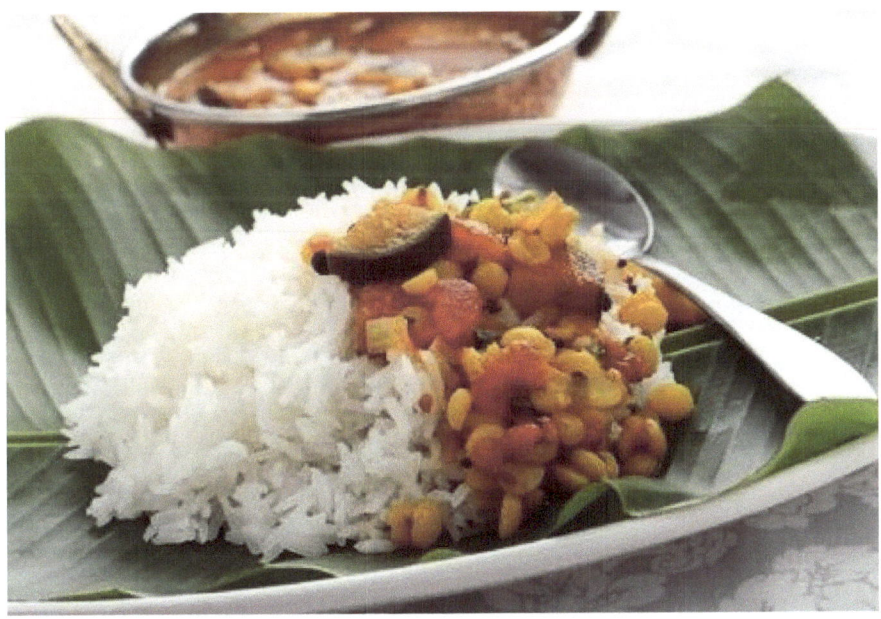

The woman of the house is going to spread the banana leaf in front of you. After that, she is going to serve rice, curry, and other dried vegetable dishes on the banana leaf. Once you are done with your meal, you are just going to roll up your leaf and throw it in the garden, where it goes back into the ecosystem.

A banana is definitely going to be part of your diet, when you are eating off this banana leaf, even today, in many parts of Southeast Asia and the Indian subcontinent, especially the states of southern India. Metal plates are only for occasions when you want to make a special splash, and the celebration is not festive. Otherwise, you just go to the market, and get a fresh supply of banana leaves. I have also drunk hot liquids in containers made up of dried banana leaves. If you are traveling somewhere in central America, your tamales are going to be served to you, hot and grilled, wrapped up in banana leaves.

Using Banana Leaves for Cooking

Banana leaves are used very often in Asian cooking, especially when you want to cook something which is normally wrapped up in parchment paper or in tinfoil. You can bake and steam meat in these banana leaves. Just get a packet of banana leaves, in your nearest Asian store-they are quite inexpensive – and use them, when you are cooking.

Remember to place these packages in a tray, or in a casserole, because if the ingredients inside are juicy, you are going to find them dripping and staining your oven.

Grilling Tip

Try out this tip, especially when you are going to grow small pieces of meat, which have this funny habit of falling through your grill rack. Place the barbecue items on a banana leaf, which you have spread on the rack. Then grill as you would grill these pieces of meat, fish, vegetables, or any other barbecue or grill item.

These leaves are going to turn dark green at first and then turned brown slowly, as they are subjected to heat. Do not worry. You are also going to find the food much tastier, thanks to the banana leaf flavor.

The banana leaves that you have bought in the supermarket can be wrapped up in plastic and put back into the freezer. You will need to defrost them before using.

Cut them with scissors to the size you want.

Using Banana Leaves for Wrapping Food and Steaming

You have the prepared food in front of you. They can be pieces of meat, shrimp, pieces of vegetable or anything else mixed with the little traditional sauce, or curry paste, just so that it is in a manageable paste/liquid form.

Cut the pieces of banana leaves, to the required size, spread them out on your kitchen counter and place the food inside. Wrap the leaf, as if you are wrapping up a handkerchief. Close the sides with toothpicks. Alternatively, you can lay the seam side portions down on the bottom of your baking tray or casserole, and bake in the oven according to the recipes.

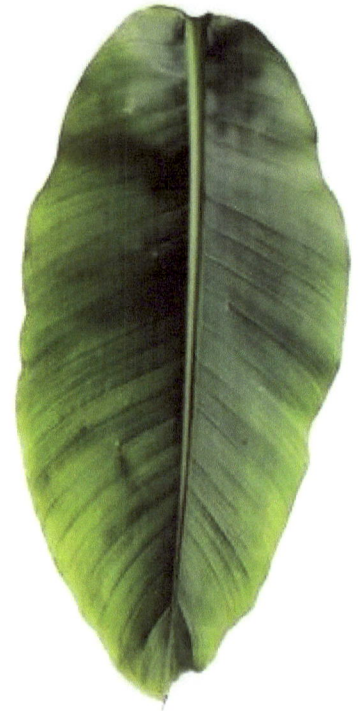

Here is an excellent way to bake fish in banana leaves. This is a recipe from Thailand.

http://thaifood.about.com/od/thairecipes/r/Salmon.htm

Banana Fiber

Did you know that banana fiber was considered to be a very valuable item to make clothing in Japan, more than 700 years ago, and much before that? The shoots as well as the leaves were cut periodically, and boiled with lye, so that the fibers could be obtained. The quality of the fibers would depend on the age of the shoots and the leaves. These fibers could then be spun into clothes. Kimonos would be made from the inner fibers and outer fibers which were coarser in texture could be made into tablecloths.

All this, including weaving of clothes has been a part of Japanese culture and proud tradition for centuries. The same method of fiber extraction in Nepal is utilized to extract fiber from the stem and the trunk of the banana tree. After the fiber has been extracted, and collected, it is sent to Kathmandu where it is woven into traditional Nepali clothing and rugs. These are amazingly soft, and you can buy them certified with an inspected for top-quality "RugMark" stamp.

When I was living in the south of India as a child, I saw a friend's mother gathering fresh jasmine flowers from her garden every morning. This is part of South Indian tradition where the ladies of the house, make flower garlands every day from Jasmine for their hair and for all the female members of the family, and even their neighbor's children!

Instead of using cotton thread, she used banana fiber thread, like her ancestors had done down the centuries. The garlands did not break, even though I as well as her daughter were quite firm believers in the tomboyish art of rough-and-tumble, even though her mother believed in girls –will- be- girls and sent us out with Jasmine flower garlands in our hair, when she shooed us out outdoors.

Banana and Coconut Rings with Palm Sugar

This is an amazingly unusual taste, where you are going to be wrapping up bananas in a covering of boiled rice.

But before you make this dish, you need to know how to make coconut milk.

Coconut Milk and Coconut Cream

You can buy this in the market, but it is better to make this at home, with some desiccated coconut. Coconut milk is not the liquid product, which you find inside the coconut. That is coconut water. Place 2 cups of desiccated coconut in a large bowl. Cover with 2 ½ cups of boiling hot water. Cover the bowl, and allow to stand until the mixture is warm.

Mix this with your hand, then strain the liquid as well as the coconut through a cloth, or a fine mesh, squeezing out as much of coconut milk as you can. This is going to give you about one and a half cups of thick milk. You can use this liquid, whenever any recipe calls for coconut milk or coconut cream.

You can use the desiccated coconut again by adding another 2 ½ cups of water. Water and continue as the valve you are going to get a more dilute and watery milk. You can combine this and watery milk with the first thicker milk and use this as a good substitute for the canned coconut milk, which you buy in the market.

You can also blend them, and process them together for 20 seconds, then strain and use.

Now we are going to take **one and a half cups of coconut milk, 2/3 cups of short grain rice, and two large bananas.**

The **palm sugar sauce** is going to be made of ¾ cups of palm sugar, 1 ½ cups of coconut cream and ¾ cup of water.

Pour the coconut milk into a saucepan. Bring it to a boil. Add the rice, and reduce the. Simmer, partly covered over very low heat, stirring continuously for about 15 minutes. The rice is going to be tender, and all the coconut milk will have been absorbed. Allow to stand for 10 minutes.

Spread the rice mixture onto a sheet of plastic wrap. Spread the mixture around each banana until the bananas are enclosed completely.

Wrap the bananas in the plastic wrap and refrigerate overnight.

Unwrap the bananas and cut into thick slices. Make the palm sugar sauce by combining the sugar as well as the water in a saucepan and stirring "heat until the sugar has been dissolved. Bring this sugar to a boil and boil the syrup uncovered for two minutes. Remove the sugar syrup from the heat and stir in the coconut cream.

Serve the sliced bananas with warm sauce and any other fruit. If you want, you can chill this again before serving.

Plantain and Lamb Curry

This is a traditional curry, which is normally made up of lamb mixed with plantains.

For this, you need

400 g of boned lamb

One Plantain peeled and chopped into small pieces

four teaspoonfuls of a good cooking oil.

1 teaspoon mustard seeds, 2 ½ cm fresh ginger root, chopped

Five cloves of garlic.

Three Sliced tomatoes

Two green chilies and 10 curry leaves

The spices you are going to use are half a teaspoon each of coriander seeds, ground turmeric and chili powder. Salt to taste.

Heat the oil in your Wok. Add the mustard seeds and fry until they start to pop. Add the curry leaves, then. After that, add the green chilies, garlic, and the ginger, and sauté over medium heat for three minutes. Add the onions and cook for another 10 minutes under the onions are slightly golden brown.

Stir in the coriander, turmeric, tomatoes and chili powder and mix them well. Then add the lamb and fry for three minutes, until the spices are incorporated in the meat. Then add 400 mL of water. Allow to boil, then cover and cook for 15 minutes over low heat.

Mix the salt with the plantain pieces. Add to the cooking lamb. Allow to cook for another 15 minutes until the plantain is tender and the Lamb is cooked thoroughly.

Serve hot with rice.

Banana Bread

1 ¾ cup sifted all-purpose flour

2 teaspoon baking powder

¼ teaspoon baking soda

Half teaspoon salt

2/3 cup sugar

1/3 cup butter or shortening

Two eggs unbeaten.

Half a cup of chopped nuts

1 cup mashed ripe bananas.

Set the oven at 350°F to preheat.

Grease a 9 x 5 x 3 loaf pan. Sift the baking powder, flour, salt and soda together.

Cream the shortening, eggs and sugar in your blender for three minutes.

Add the banana, nuts, and the flour mixture in your shortening mixture and beat until it is smooth. This is going to take about one minute. Remember to scrape the bowl if the mixture sticks to the sides.

Turn into the pan and bake for one hour or until done. Cool on the cake rack. Store it overnight before slicing.

Conclusion

For those interested in making banana chips, here is a URL

http://www.youtube.com/watch?v=5f3fj4Z0-o8

You can also fry them, as it is done traditionally, in Jamaica

http://www.youtube.com/watch?v=Z42plN4JeZU

This book has given you a lot of information on bananas, along with its value as a food, and also as a healing agent. Remember not to eat bananas, when they have become overripe and the fruit flies are more interested in them, than you are. Those are the bananas which are normally used for medicinal purposes, because overripe bananas with milk can help healing your stomach.

However, if you are healthy, just pick two firm bananas, which do not feel like they are mashed enough to baby food consistency and enjoy!

Live long and prosper!

Author Bio

Dueep Jyot Singh is a Management and IT Professional who managed to gather Postgraduate qualifications in Management and English and Degrees in Science, French and Education while pursuing different enjoyable career options like being an hospital administrator, IT,SEO and HRD Database Manager/ trainer, movie scriptwriter, theatre artiste and public speaker, lecturer in French, Marketing and Advertising, ex-Editor of Hearts On Fire (now known as Solstice) Books Missouri USA, advice columnist and cartoonist, publisher and Aviation School trainer, ex- moderator on Medico.in, banker, student councilor ,travelogue writer … among other things! One fine morning, she decided that she had enough of killing herself by Degrees and went back to her first love -- writing. It's more enjoyable! She already has 48 published academic and 14 fiction- in- different- genre books under her belt.

When she is not designing websites or making Graphic design illustrations for clients , she is browsing through old bookshops hunting for treasures, of which she has an enviable collection – including R.L. Stevenson, O.Henry, Dornford Yates, Maurice Walsh, C.N.Williamson, Sapper, Bartimeus and the crown of her collection-Dickens "The Old Curiosity Shop," and so on… Just call her "Renaissance Woman" - collecting herbal remedies, acting like Universal Helping Hand/Agony Aunt, or escaping to her dear mountains for a bit of exploring, collecting herbs and plants, and trekking.

Check out some of the other JD-Biz Publishing books

Health Learning Series

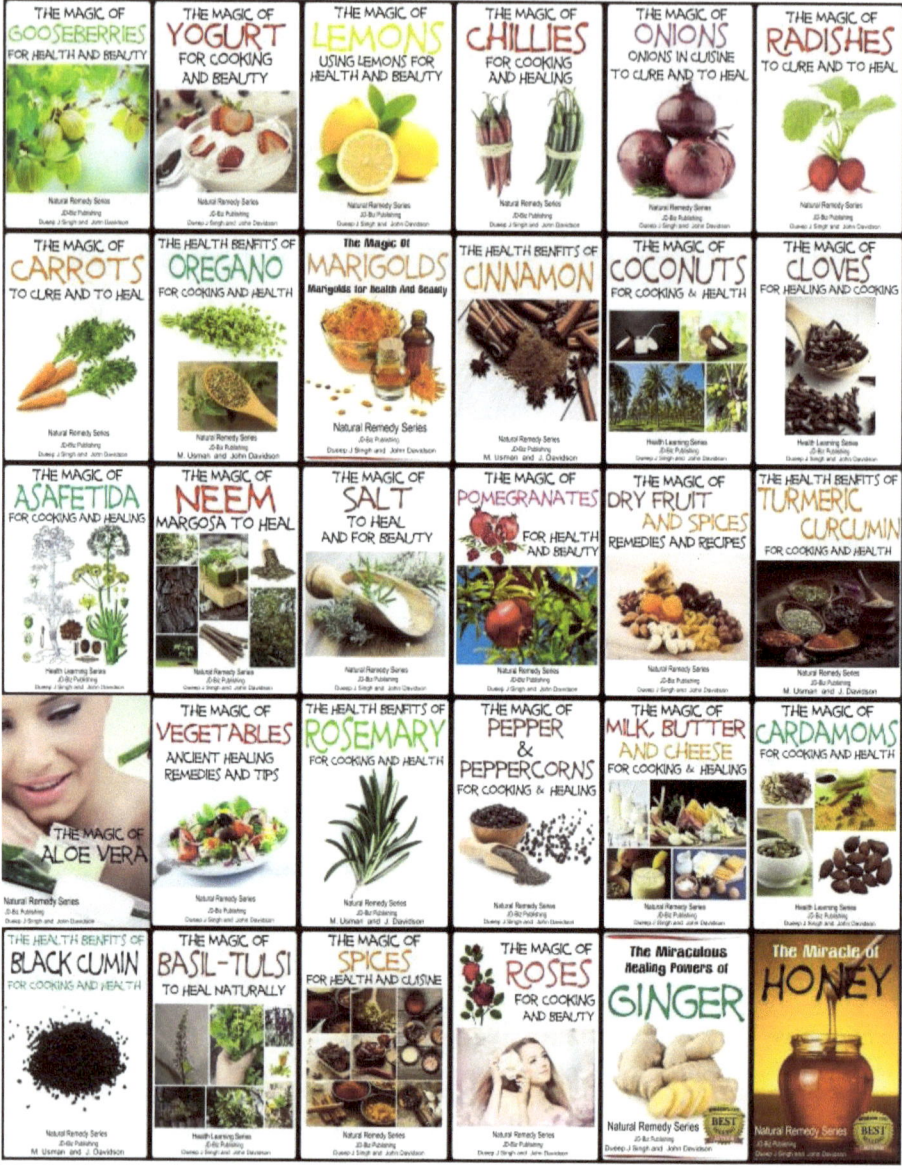

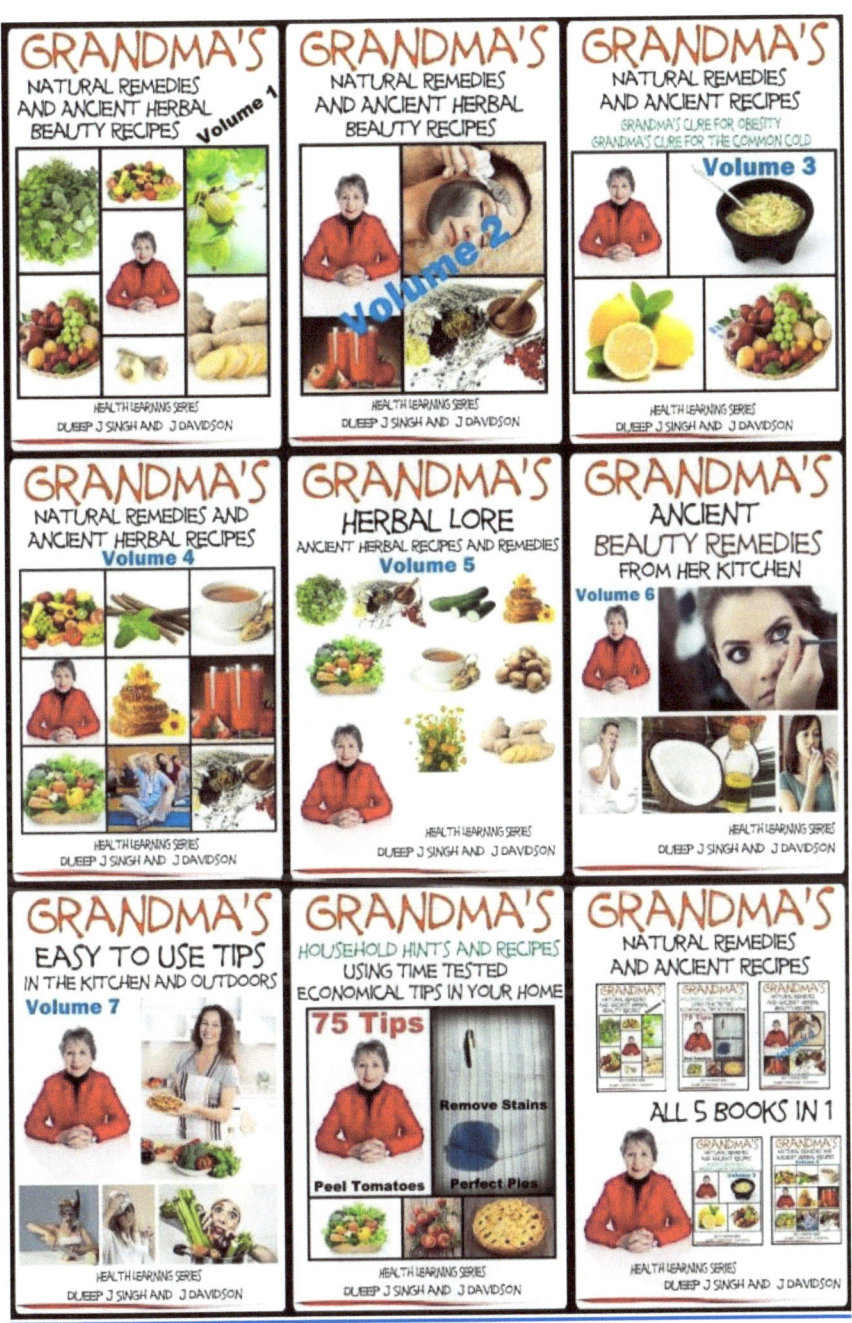

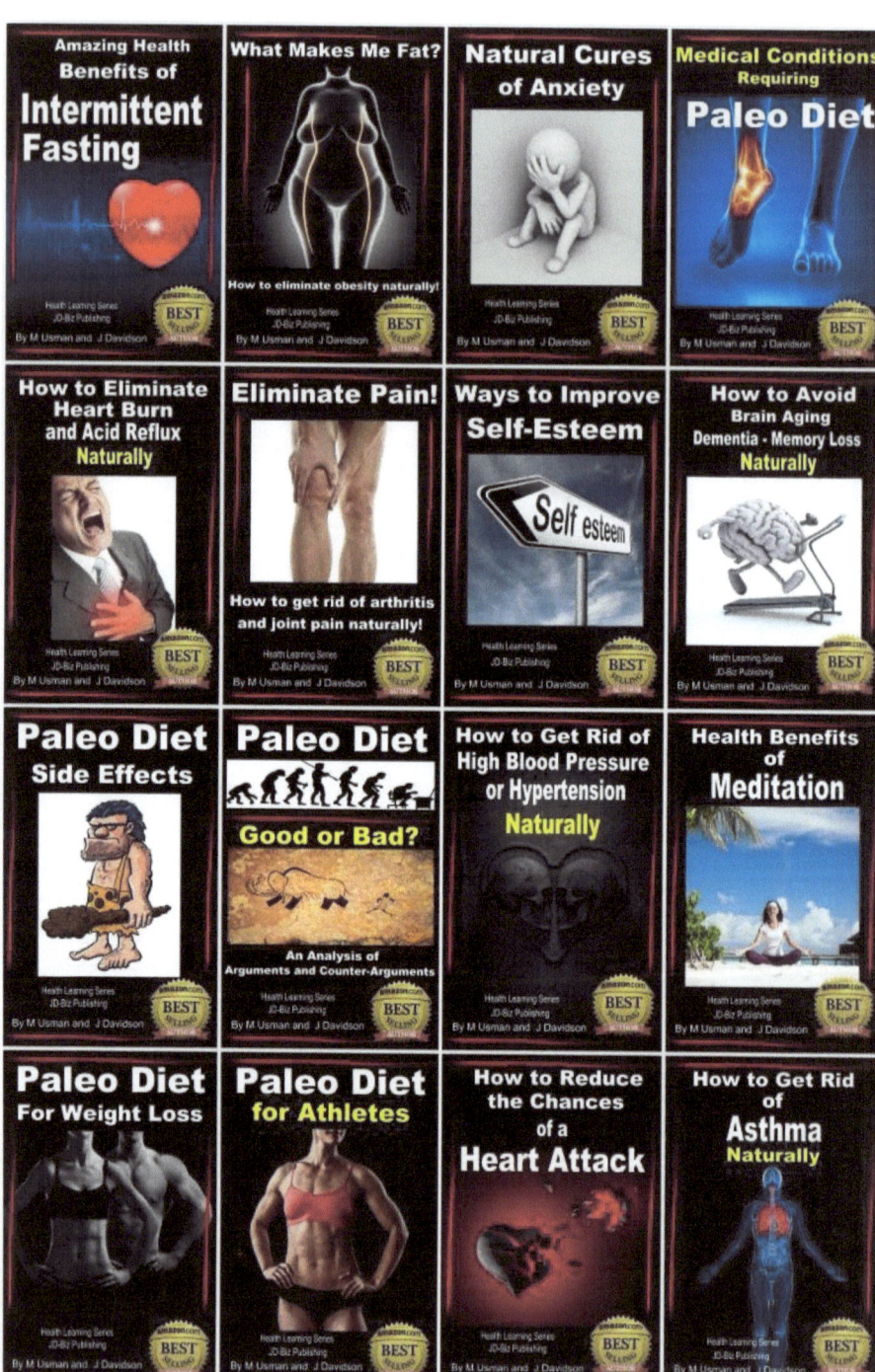

Amazing Animal Book Series

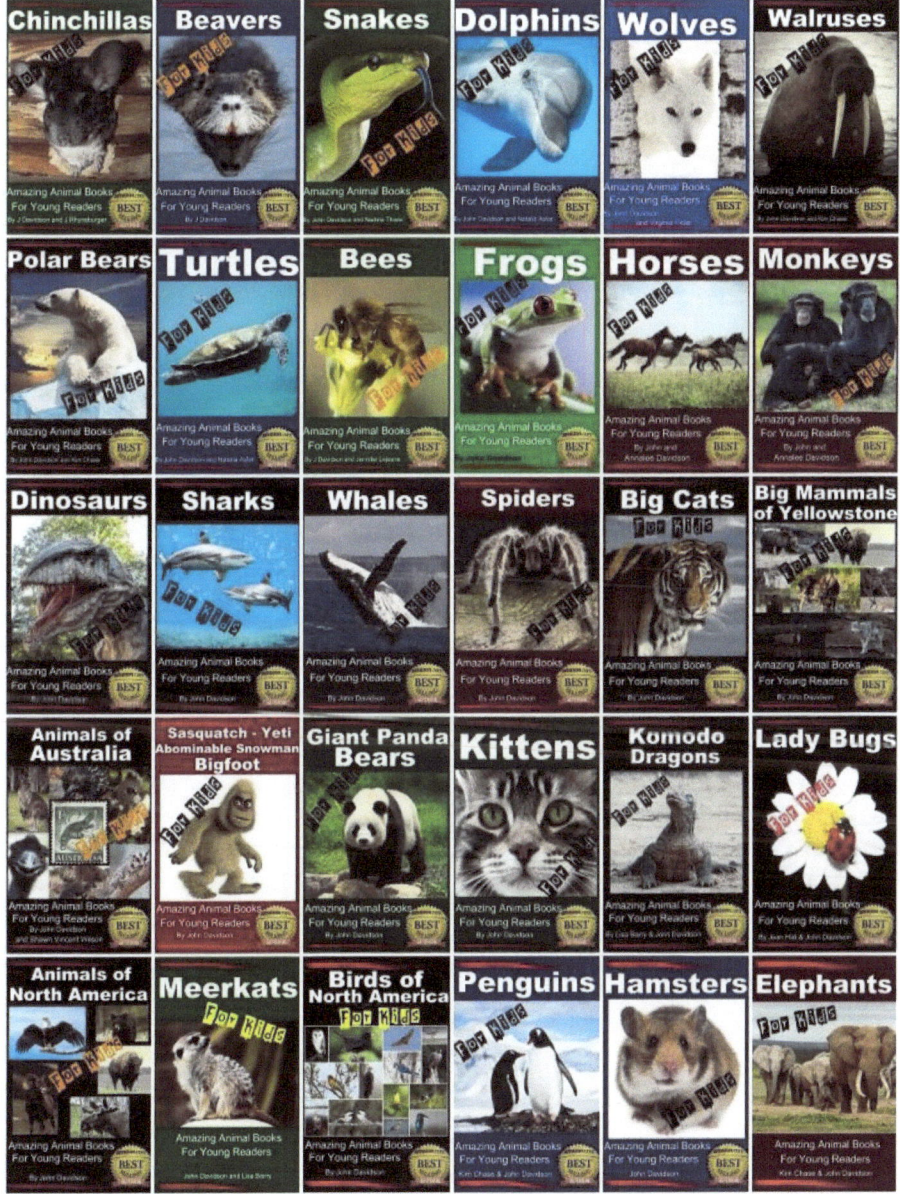

Learn To Draw Series

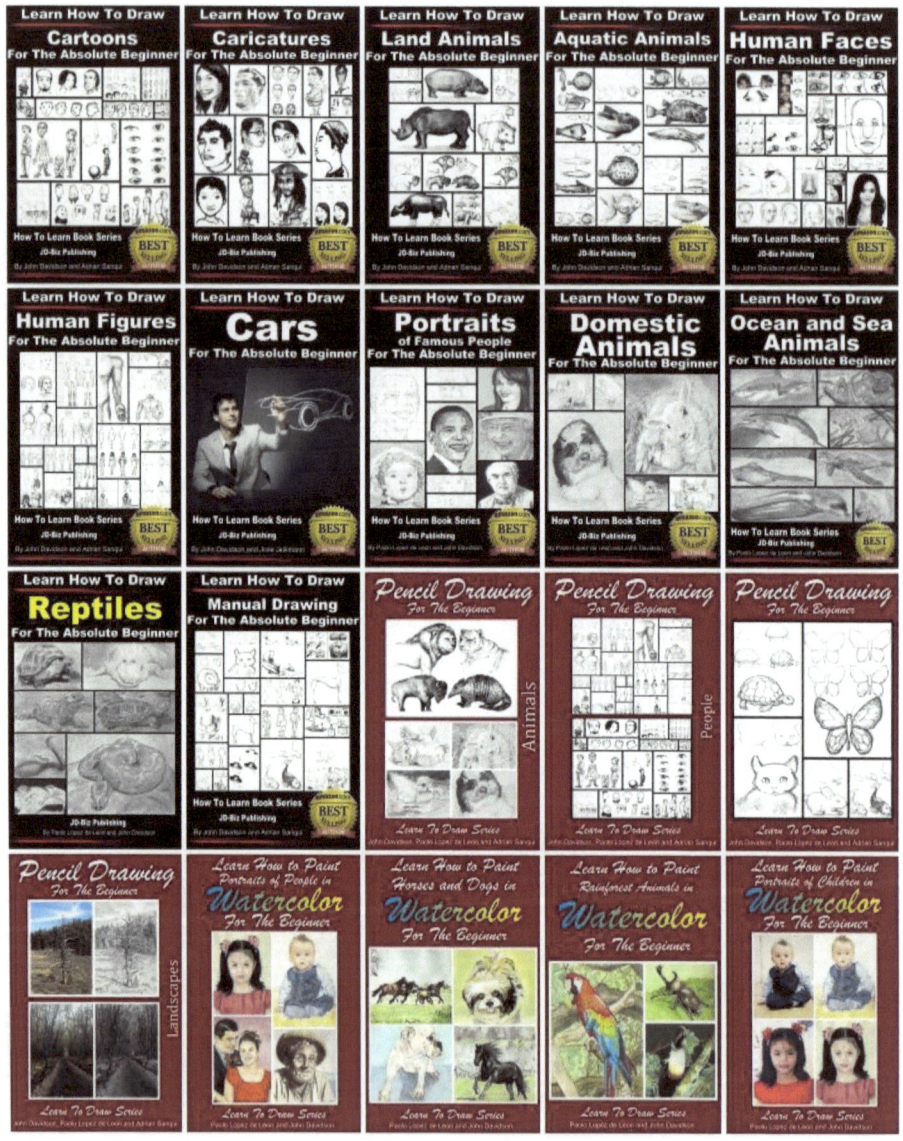

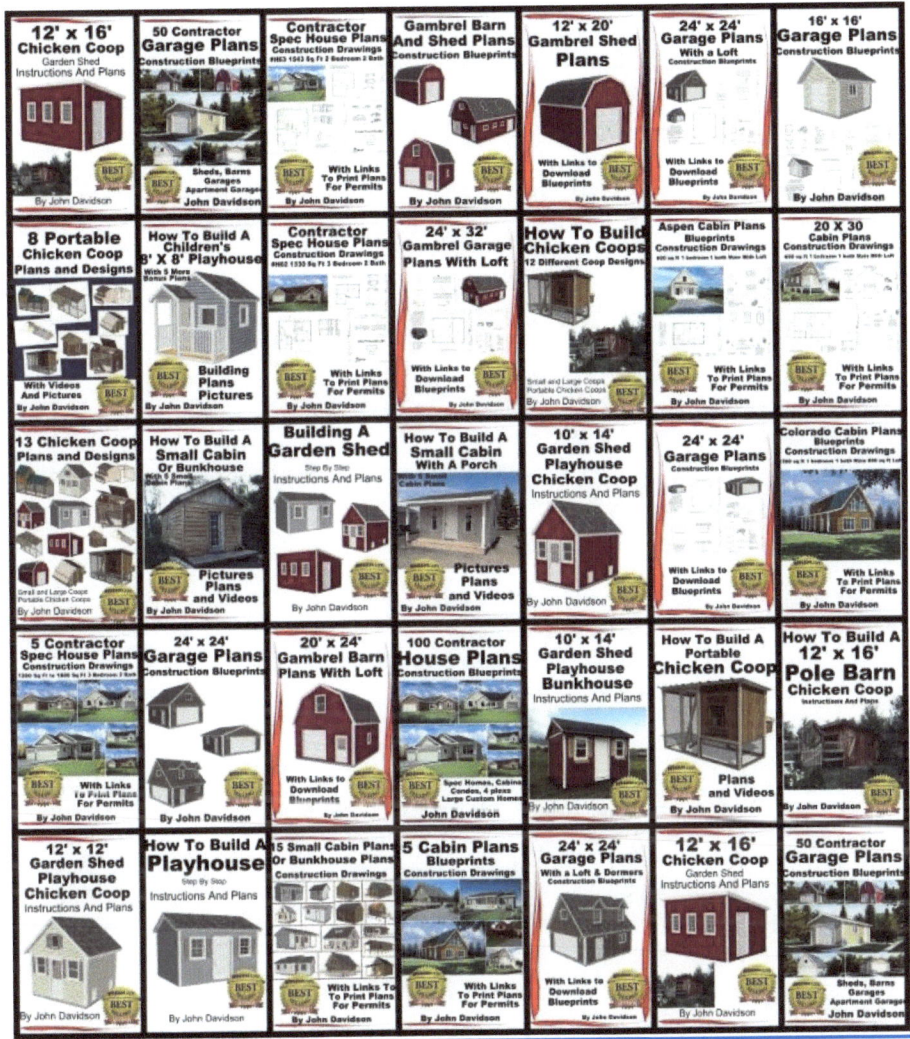

Entrepreneur Book Series

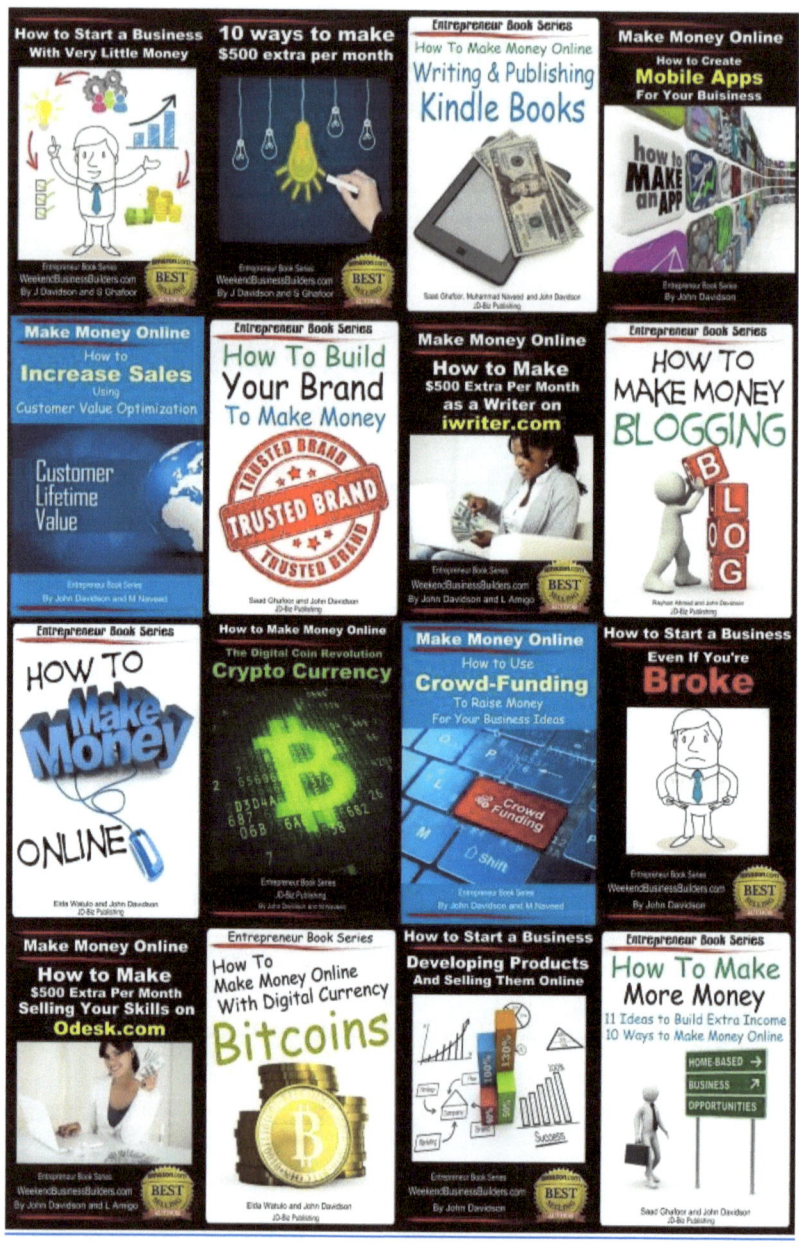

Our books are available at

1. Amazon.com

2. Barnes and Noble

3. Itunes

4. Kobo

5. Smashwords

6. Google Play Books

Download Free Books!

http://MendonCottageBooks.com

Publisher

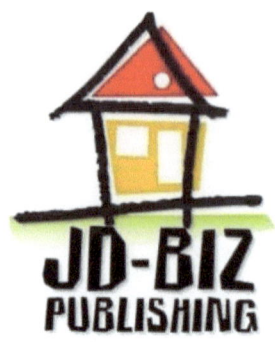

JD-Biz Corp

P O Box 374

Mendon, Utah 84325

http://www.jd-biz.com/

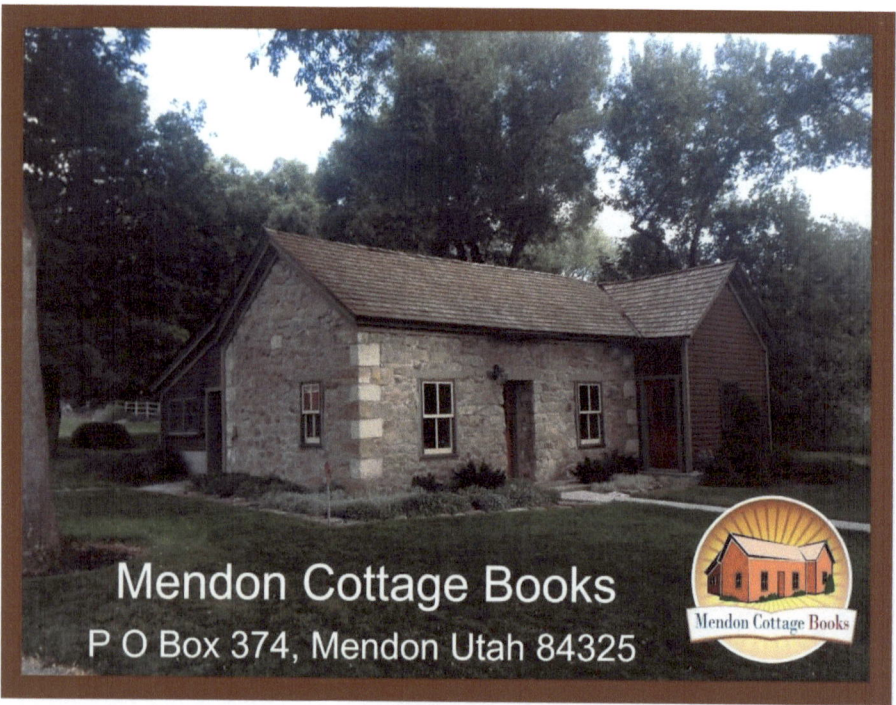

Mendon Cottage Books

P O Box 374, Mendon Utah 84325